Simple Gout Exercise For Senior

Optimizing Joint Health With A Comprehensive Guide for Seniors with Gout.

TABLE OF CONTENT

INTRODUCTION

Seniors who suffer from gout, a complicated form of arthritis, may experience major difficulties in their daily lives. Although it is frequently related to food decisions, the therapy for this condition encompasses more than just dietary restrictions. The purpose of this introduction is to offer a complete review of gout in younger adults and to highlight the critical role that physical activity plays in the management of this condition.

Understanding Gout in Seniors

A kind of inflammatory arthritis called gout is typified by the accumulation of uric acid crystals in the joints, which causes discomfort, edema, and inflammation. Although it can afflict people of any age, elderly people are more vulnerable because of things like altered metabolism with aging and a higher chance of coexisting illnesses.

Gout frequently appears in older adults' big toes, knees, wrists, and elbows. Gout episodes can cause excruciating pain that affects one's mobility and general quality of life. Customizing successful management techniques for gout requires an understanding of the unique obstacles faced by seniors.

Seniors who acquire gout are susceptible to several conditions. Age-related changes in renal function can lead to a reduction in the excretion of uric acid, which can exacerbate its buildup in the joints. Seniors may also have additional medical illnesses like diabetes or hypertension, which can make managing their gout more difficult and worsen its symptoms.

Elderly people and those who care for them must identify gout symptoms as soon as possible. These might include warmth in the afflicted region, edema, redness, and abrupt, severe joint pain. To lessen the negative effects of gout on the joint health of elders, early diagnosis and treatment are essential.

Risk Factors for Gout in Seniors

It is essential to comprehend the risk factors linked to gout in seniors to avoid and treat the condition. In addition to heredity, gender (men are more sensitive), certain drugs, and lifestyle choices, age itself is a risk factor. Gout is mostly caused by dietary practices, especially consuming alcohol and foods high in purines.

Impact of Gout on Seniors' Quality of Life

Beyond the obvious physical symptoms, gout can significantly affect seniors' general health and day-to-day activities. Their quality of life might be further compromised by anxiety and despair brought on by chronic pain and the worry of more episodes. Seniors' capacity to carry out daily tasks may be restricted, which may have an impact on their independence and social interaction.

Diagnostic Approaches for Gout in Seniors

Laboratory testing, clinical examination, and medical history assessment are all used in the diagnosis of gout in the elderly. In addition to using blood tests to detect uric acid levels, healthcare practitioners may still use joint aspiration to investigate synovial fluid as a conclusive diagnostic technique. When diagnosing an elderly patient, it may be necessary to carefully take into account any pre-existing medical issues and any drug interactions.

Importance of Exercise in Gout Management

Gout management in older adults involves more than just taking medicine and making adjustments to one's diet; it also involves taking a comprehensive approach that includes engaging in regular physical activity. In the prevention and therapy of a wide range of health issues, exercise is an essential component, and gout is neither an exception nor an exception. People who are elderly, on the other hand, could be concerned and hesitant about participating in physical activities because they are afraid of their gout symptoms becoming worse.

- **Benefits of Exercise for Seniors with Gout**

Seniors who are controlling their gout might get a plethora of benefits from engaging in regular and adequate physical activity. To begin, it assists in the preservation of joint flexibility and range of motion, hence lowering the likelihood of experiencing the stiffness and discomfort that are associated with gout episodes. The second benefit of exercise is that it helps with weight control, which is an essential component of gout care because the presence of excess weight can lead to increased levels of uric acid.

Additionally, physical activity is beneficial to cardiovascular health, which is a facet of gout care that is sometimes neglected. Comorbid diseases, such as hypertension and cardiovascular disease, are more likely to be present in elderly patients who suffer from recurrent gout. The practice of cardiovascular workouts not only helps to maintain a healthy heart generally, but it also has the potential to enhance circulation, which in turn can facilitate the elimination of uric acid crystals from joints.

- **Considerations Before Starting an Exercise Routine**

Even though exercise is healthy, older citizens who suffer from gout should approach it with caution and under the supervision of licensed medical specialists. Some of the things that should be taken into consideration are the type and intensity of activity, any joint injury that may already be present, and the general health state. Before beginning any kind of workout plan, older citizens should discuss it with their healthcare physician to make certain that it is suitable for their specific requirements and the symptoms they are now experiencing.

- **Types of Exercises for Gout Management**

It is crucial for the long-term success of seniors who suffer from gout to modify their exercise routines so that they are suitable for their demands and restrictions. While walking, swimming, and gentle stretching are all examples of low-impact workouts, they are perfect for preserving joint health since they do not place an excessive amount of stress on joints that are already weak. It is possible to offer additional support to joints through the use of strengthening exercises that target main muscle groups. This can help reduce the risk of problems connected to gout.

CHAPTER ONE: BASICS OF GOUT

Gout is a kind of arthritis that has been identified for ages. It is frequently linked to lavish food and certain indulgences that are associated with royal lifestyles. However, its origins go beyond the decisions that people make about their nutrition, and they include intricate metabolic processes as well as genetic predispositions. Gout is examined in this chapter, which dives into the principles of the condition, including what it is, the numerous variables that contribute to its development, and how it presents itself in older people.

What is Gout?

Urate crystals depositing in the joints are a characteristic of gout, a kind of inflammatory arthritis. Hyperuricemia, or too much uric acid in the blood, is the condition that causes these crystals to develop. Purines are naturally occurring substances found in certain foods and are broken down by the body to produce uric acid as a byproduct.

Uric acid dissolves in blood, travels through the kidneys, and is eliminated in urine in a healthy person. But when uric acid is produced in excess or the kidneys are unable to properly excrete it, urate crystals build up in the joints, causing inflammation and the telltale signs of gout.

Types of Gout

Understanding the many manifestations of gout is essential for precise diagnosis and treatment. Acute and chronic gout are the two main kinds of gout.

- Acute gout is characterized by sudden and severe joint pain, swelling, redness, and tenderness. The attacks usually happen at night and can be caused by things like alcohol, particular meals, or anxiety.

- Chronic Gout: If gout is not successfully controlled, it can develop into chronic gout. Individuals with chronic gout may endure recurring gout episodes, as well as joint degeneration. Chronic gout requires regular

treatment to avoid long-term consequences.

Gout in Seniors

Gout is more likely to affect elderly people than younger people because of the changes that occur in metabolism and renal function as people get older. Because of the natural process of aging, the kidneys may become less effective in eliminating uric acid, which can result in a buildup of the substance in the circulation. Additionally, older adults may be more likely to suffer from other health issues, such as diabetes or hypertension, which can have a role in the development of gout or the worsening of its symptoms.

Causes and Risk Factors

For both the prevention of gout and its efficient management, it is vital to have a solid understanding of the causes and risk factors linked with the condition. While certain aspects of one's lifestyle may be altered by the implementation of positive adjustments, others, such as heredity, are beyond the control of the individual.

- **Dietary Choices**

In the development of gout, diet is a crucial factor that plays a big influence. It is possible for raised uric acid levels to be caused by foods that are high in purines. Some examples of such foods are red meat, organ meats, shellfish, and some vegetables such include asparagus and mushrooms. In addition, there is a correlation between excessive alcohol use, particularly beer and spirits, and an increased chance of developing gout.

- **Genetics**

The likelihood of an individual developing gout can be affected by several genetic variables. There is a possibility that the probability of acquiring gout is increased if there is a history of the ailment in the member's family. Additionally, how the body processes and removes uric acid might be influenced by genetic variables.

- **Medical Conditions**

Several medical factors might make the likelihood of acquiring gout higher. Chronic illnesses such as hypertension, diabetes, and metabolic syndrome are examples of disorders that can have a role in the development of gout or the worsening of its symptoms. It is also possible for medications like aspirin and diuretics to cause a rise in uric acid levels.

- **Obesity**

A key risk factor for gout is having an excessive amount of body fat. There is a correlation between obesity and both an increase in the generation of uric acid and a decrease in the kidneys' ability to excrete it. Since this is the case, weight control is an essential component of both the prevention and therapy of gout.

- **Age and Gender**

Gout is more common in those who are older, and the chance of developing the condition increases with age. In general, males are more likely to suffer from gout than women; however, postmenopausal women are at a higher risk of developing the condition compared to premenopausal women.

Symptoms and Diagnosis

Gout is a condition that requires rapid diagnosis and treatment, thus it is crucial to recognize the signs of gout. The bouts of gout frequently come on unexpectedly and can be quite severe, necessitating prompt medical intervention.

- **Symptoms of Gout**

Gout is characterized by the abrupt onset of excruciating pain, usually in the joints. The afflicted joint turns red, swollen, and incredibly sensitive to pressure. Gout attacks can be brought on by stress, specific meals, alcohol intake, or other circumstances. They typically happen at night.

The big toe, ankle, knee, and joints in the hands and wrists are among the joints that are frequently impacted. Even the slightest touch or the weight of a bedsheet can be quite uncomfortable due to the severe nature of the pain.

- **Complications of Untreated Gout**

Gout can have side effects, such as tophi development if it is not treated. Urate crystal lumps, known as tophi, can grow under the skin and around joints, deforming the body. Reduced range of motion and joint degeneration are further consequences of chronic gout.

- **Diagnostic Approaches for Gout**

Diagnosing gout includes a mix of clinical examination, medical history assessment, and laboratory studies.

- Clinical Evaluation: Medical professionals will evaluate the patient's symptoms, taking into account the joint involvement pattern, the location and degree of pain, and any aggravating factors.

- Evaluation of Medical History: Determining risk factors and possible gout causes is made easier with a comprehensive medical history. A person's food habits, medical history, and current health are taken into account.

- Laboratory Testing: Uric acid levels are frequently determined by blood tests. It's crucial to remember that high uric acid levels by themselves do not always indicate gout; some people who have high levels may never get gout, while other people who have gout may have normal uric acid levels.

- Joint Aspiration: A method in which synovial fluid is extracted from the afflicted joint, joint aspiration is used by medical professionals to make a conclusive diagnosis of gout. The diagnosis is supported by the fluid's urate crystal presence.

Differential Diagnosis

Other types of arthritis, such as rheumatoid arthritis and osteoarthritis, frequently exhibit symptoms that are similar to those of gout. When it comes to ensuring suitable and successful therapy, differential diagnosis is necessary. The evaluation of joint damage and the elimination of other problems may be accomplished via the utilization of imaging tests such as X-rays or ultrasounds.

CHAPTER TWO: EXERCISE AND GOUT

Physical activity is an essential component in the treatment of a wide range of health issues, and gout is not an exception to this rule. Although older citizens who suffer from gout can be reluctant to participate in physical activities out of the worry that their symptoms will become worse, a well-designed exercise plan can bring about a multitude of advantages. This chapter discusses the significance of physical activity for elderly people who suffer from gout, the factors to take into account before beginning an exercise regimen, and the numerous types of exercises that are specifically designed to be useful in managing gout.

Benefits of Exercise for Seniors with Gout

The benefits of regular, safe exercise for elders with gout are numerous. Despite popular belief, physical activity can be an effective means of preventing and controlling gout symptoms.

- **Maintaining Joint Flexibility and Range of Motion**

Regular exercise contributes to the preservation of joint range of motion and flexibility. This is especially crucial for gout sufferers because stiffness and decreased movement are frequent side effects both during and after gout episodes. To improve flexibility and prevent joint stiffness, try some gentle stretching exercises.

- **Weight Management**

Being overweight significantly increases your chances of developing gout. Obesity is linked to decreased renal excretion as well as increased uric acid synthesis. Frequent exercise helps seniors reach and maintain a healthy weight by aiding in weight management. Thus, uric acid levels may be lowered, and gout episodes may occur less frequently and with less intensity.

- **Cardiovascular Health**

Gouty seniors are frequently more susceptible to heart disease and other cardiovascular diseases including hypertension. Cardiovascular workouts, including swimming, cycling, or walking, enhance circulation in addition to supporting heart health in general. Increased blood flow helps to control gout by assisting in the elimination of uric acid crystals from joints.

- **Strengthening Muscles and Joints**

Exercises aimed at strengthening the main muscle groups provide gout-affected joints more support. Robust muscles contribute to joint stabilization, lowering the chance of injury and promoting general joint health. For seniors treating gout, resistance exercise might be very helpful when adapted appropriately for their specific needs.

- **Mood and Well-being**

Exercise regularly is shown to improve mood and general wellbeing. Gouty seniors may suffer from anxiety and despair as a result of their ongoing pain and worry about future episodes. Exercise releases endorphins, which are the body's natural mood enhancers and can lead to a happier perspective and better mental health.

- **Improved Sleep Quality**

Sleep habits can be disturbed by gout episodes, which are marked by excruciating pain. Frequent exercise has been demonstrated to enhance the quality of sleep, which is essential for general health and wellbeing. Seniors with gout might improve their sleep hygiene by starting a regular exercise regimen.

- **Social Engagement**

When you take part in group workout activities or programs, you get the opportunity to engage with other people. The mental and emotional well-being of elders needs to participate in social activities. When you connect with other people who have health challenges that are similar to your own, you may create an environment that is encouraging and helpful.

Considerations Before Starting an Exercise Routine

Although seniors who suffer from gout may reap the advantages of exercise, there are a few things that need to be taken into mind before beginning an exercise regimen. When it comes to ensuring that exercise makes a good contribution to the management of gout, safety, and customized techniques are of the utmost importance.

- **Consultation with Healthcare Provider.**

Before beginning any fitness plan, seniors with gout should contact their doctor. This is especially crucial if you have any pre-existing health issues or are concerned about potential drug interactions. Healthcare practitioners can advise on the type and intensity of exercise that is most appropriate for each individual's needs.

- **Understanding Joint Health.**

Seniors with gout may have joint damage or deformities as a result of recurring bouts. Understanding the exact state of their joints is critical for designing an activity regimen that reduces the risk of worsening symptoms. Low-impact activities are commonly suggested to protect fragile joints.

- **Gradual progression.**

Seniors who have been sedentary for a time or are new to fitness should aim for steady development. Beginning with low-intensity exercises and gradually increasing length and intensity helps the body to adapt while reducing the danger of damage. Patience and persistence are essential for creating a sustainable training habit.

- **Pain Monitoring**

While some discomfort when activity is typical, seniors who have gout should monitor their pain levels. If joint pain persists beyond the normal discomfort associated with exercise, it's time to reconsider your exercise program and talk with a healthcare specialist.

- **Hydration and Nutrition**

Proper hydration is vital for gout sufferers because it assists in the removal of uric acid. Seniors who exercise should keep hydrated. Maintaining a balanced diet, with a focus on purine-rich foods, also helps with gout treatment.

- **Individual Preferences and Limitations**

Adherence to a fitness plan requires taking into account individual preferences and limits. Seniors are more inclined to persist with activities that they like. Tailoring workouts to meet any physical limits or preferences improves the chances of long-term adherence.

Types of Exercises for Gout Management

To effectively treat gout through exercise, it is necessary to engage in a variety of activities, each of which has a distinct function in enhancing joint health and general well-being.

- **Low-Impact Exercises**

Low-impact workouts are extremely soft on the joints and are especially well-suited for older citizens who suffer from gout disease. Participating in these exercises helps to preserve joint flexibility and cardiovascular health without putting an excessive amount of stress on joints that are already fragile. The following are some examples of low-impact exercises:

- Walking is an easy and efficient method to work your heart out without putting too much strain on your joints.

- Swimming or water aerobics: The buoyancy of the water gives you a full-body exercise while minimizing the strain on your joints.

- Cycling: Cycling, whether inside or outdoors, is a low-impact activity that improves cardiovascular health.

Stretching and Flexibility Exercises

For elderly gout sufferers, maintaining joint flexibility is essential. Frequent stretching exercises improve the range of motion and lessen the chance of gout attack-related stiffness. Among the many ways to include stretching in your everyday practice are:

- Yoga: This kind of physical and mental well-being combines mindfulness with moderate stretching.
- Tai Chi: Slow, deliberate motions are used in this age-old Chinese martial art to enhance joint health, flexibility, and balance.

Strengthening Exercises

Strengthening exercises focus on the main muscle groups, giving gout-affected joints more support. Resistant activities can be incorporated into strength training, but it's necessary to proceed cautiously, particularly if joint injury already exists. Exercises for strengthening include, for example:

Bodyweight Workouts: Without the need for further equipment, squats, lunges, and wall push-ups are efficient bodyweight exercises that build muscle.

Resistance Training: With little to no strain on joints, using resistance bands or small weights can assist in strengthening particular muscle groups.

Range of Motion Exercises

Preventing stiffness and enhancing general joint health requires maintaining a wide range of motion in the joints. Exercises for a range of motion might include:

- Joint Circles: To preserve flexibility, make light circular motions with your ankles, knees, wrists, and shoulders.
- Dynamic Stretching: It might be helpful to include stretches that involve actively engaging muscles throughout their whole range of motion.

Balance and Stability Exercises

Exercises for stability and balance are essential for preventing falls, particularly in older adults. While considering joint health, some exercises that enhance balance include:

- Standing on One Leg: This easy workout enhances stability and balance.
- Balance Exercises on Stable Surfaces: You may improve stability without overstressing your joints by using stability balls or balancing pads.

CHAPTER THREE: TAILORING EXERCISES FOR SENIORS

A strategy that is intelligent and tailored, taking into consideration elements such as joint health, mobility, and general well-being, is required to tailor workouts for patients who are senior citizens. In this chapter, we discuss the significance of distinguishing between low-impact and high-impact exercises, the customization of exercise plans to meet the specific requirements of each individual, and the collaborative role that healthcare professionals play in guiding senior citizens toward an exercise routine that is both safe and effective.

Low-Impact vs. High-Impact Exercises

Knowing the difference between low-impact and high-impact activities is important when designing an exercise program for seniors, especially those who are managing illnesses like gout. The choice of exercise relies on an individual's fitness level, joint health, and personal preferences. Each form of exercise has advantages and disadvantages.

Low-Impact Exercises

Low-impact workouts are especially beneficial for older adults and people with gout since they are easy on the joints. These workouts improve cardiovascular health without overstressing joints that are already fragile. Let's look at some senior-specific low-impact exercises:

- Walking is an easy-to-start, low-impact activity that improves cardiovascular health without straining the joints. Seniors who walk every day might progressively increase the length of their walks as their stamina increases.

- Swimming: Two great low-impact workouts are swimming and water aerobics. Water's buoyancy works the entire body while lessening the strain on joints. Gout sufferers might benefit most from water workouts since they provide mobility without putting undue strain on their joints.

- Cycling: Cycling, whether inside or outdoors, is a low-impact activity that improves cardiovascular health. Seniors can ride in a park or on a stationary bike, varying the intensity according to their comfort level.

- Elliptical Training: Compared to jogging, the elliptical machine offers a low-impact exercise option. Seniors may use it since it mimics the motion of jogging or walking without the strain on their joints.

- Tai Chi: This traditional Chinese martial technique improves flexibility, balance, and general well-being via slow, deliberate motions. Low-impact tai chi exercises may be modified to suit different levels of fitness.

- Yoga: A great low-impact workout for elders, yoga combines mindfulness with gentle stretching. It encourages relaxation, increases flexibility, and can be modified to suit a range of skill levels.

High-Impact Exercises

High-impact activities can still be incorporated with careful thought and adaptation, even though low-impact exercises are typically advised for seniors and individuals with joint problems. Exercises with a high impact level need more power and may strain joints more. Seniors who participate in high-impact workouts should proceed with caution and seek advice from medical specialists. High-impact workout examples are as follows:

- Running and jogging can be quite taxing on the joints, but they offer vigorous cardiovascular exercise. If seniors are avid runners, they may want to think about less impactful options like elliptical machines or moderate strolling.

- Jumping jacks: Although they improve cardiovascular fitness, jumping jacks cause repeated joint trauma. Changes like low-impact jumping jacks or other aerobic substitutes could be more appropriate.

- High-Intensity Interval Training (HIIT): HIIT exercises alternate brief bursts of vigorous exertion with relaxation intervals. Seniors should approach HIIT cautiously, taking into account lower-impact options or lowering intensity, even though it is excellent for fitness.

- Step Aerobics: Because of the strain on joints, seniors may find traditional step aerobics difficult. On the other hand, low-impact or modified step aerobics can help the cardiovascular system while putting less strain on the joints.

- Sports with sudden, fast motions, like basketball and tennis, may be quite impactful. Seniors who are interested in these activities may think about making adjustments or switching to a lower-impact activity like walking tennis or pickleball.

- Seniors should pay attention to their body' needs and select workouts based on joint health and comfort level. To attain the best possible health advantages, a well-rounded exercise regimen often includes both low-impact and, where necessary, carefully adapted high-impact exercises.

Customizing Exercise Plans for Individual Needs

A varied collection of people, senior citizens have differing degrees of physical fitness, different health issues, and different personal preferences. To guarantee that the selected activities are safe, fun, and successful in boosting general well-being, it is important to tailor exercise routines to match the specific requirements of each individual.

▪ Assessing Individual Fitness Levels

It's critical to determine a person's current fitness level before designing an exercise program. Considerations like joint health, cardiovascular fitness, strength, flexibility, and balance may be part of this evaluation. Health care providers, such as fitness specialists and physical therapists, can do evaluations to establish a starting point for creating individualized exercise regimens.

- **Addressing Joint Health and Conditions**

Joint health is a key consideration when creating personalized exercise regimens for seniors with illnesses like gout. Exercise selection should take into account the joint discomfort, stiffness, or deformities that individuals with gout may feel. It's common advice to focus on joint protection and flexibility when performing low-impact activities. Exercises tailored to the afflicted joints and adjacent muscle groups may also be used.

- **Setting Realistic Goals**

Achieving and setting attainable objectives is essential to keeping up motivation and sticking to a workout schedule. Objectives could change depending on personal preferences and health goals. A senior with gout, for instance, can establish objectives to lower the frequency of gout attacks, increase joint flexibility, or reach a healthy weight. These objectives must be clear, quantifiable, and customized to each person's talents.

- **Incorporating Variety**

A varied range of exercises is included in a well-rounded workout program to target various fitness levels. Exercises for the heart and circulatory system, muscular support and flexibility, joint mobility and fall prevention, and balance training are all included in this. Plans that are tailored to incorporate a variety of activities increase overall health benefits and maintain everyday engagement.

- **Adapting to Preferences and Lifestyle**

Customizing workout regimens also entails taking lifestyle and personal preferences into account. Seniors are more likely to continue with hobbies they find enjoyable. It may be important to emphasize walking, gardening, or cycling if an elderly person enjoys outdoor activities. A more active lifestyle is also supported by adding exercise into everyday activities like doing housework or the stairs.

- **Modifications for Special Populations**

Seniors may require special considerations, particularly if they have impairments or long-term medical issues. Developing exercise regimens specifically for unique groups necessitates skill in modifying exercises to account for restrictions and optimize advantages. Seniors with a variety of needs can benefit from the advice of healthcare experts who specialize in geriatrics or adaptive fitness when developing safe and efficient exercise regimens.

Working with a Healthcare Professional

Senior fitness programs that are specifically designed for them must work in tandem with healthcare specialists. Involving healthcare professionals in the management of gout or other health disorders guarantees that exercise regimens are in line with medical advice and improve general health.

▪ Importance of Consultation

Seniors, especially those who are treating gout, should speak with their healthcare physician before starting any kind of fitness program. A complete evaluation of the patient's health situation, the discovery of any possible contraindications, and the discussion of any particular suggestions based on the patient's unique needs may all be accomplished during this session.

- **Collaboration with Physical Therapists**

Senior fitness programs are greatly influenced by physical therapists, especially for individuals with joint problems. These experts are skilled in evaluating muscular strength, joint function, and mobility. Physical therapists can offer specialized exercises, stretches, and adaptations designed to improve general musculoskeletal health and treat gout-related issues.

- **Guidance from Fitness Experts**

When developing safe and efficient workout regimens, certified fitness professionals—such as personal trainers with experience in senior fitness—can offer invaluable advice. They may suggest adaptations, keep track of development, and guarantee that workouts are executed correctly. To keep older citizens interested and motivated, fitness professionals may also provide variations to exercises.

- **Monitoring and Adjusting Plans**

For fitness programs to continue to be successful, regular evaluations and modifications are necessary. Medical practitioners can monitor development, evaluate any shifts in a patient's condition, and adjust workout regimens as necessary. Changes can be made to progressively raise the intensity or add new exercises if joint health improves or if overall fitness changes.

- **Safety Considerations**

Health care providers make sure that exercise regimens emphasize safety, particularly for elderly patients suffering from gout. They may offer direction on proper warm-up and cool-down exercises, suggest appropriate footwear, and offer advice on ways to avoid injury or overexertion. Prioritizing safety is essential to preserving a satisfying and long-lasting workout experience.

CHAPTER FOUR: SIMPLE GOUT EXERCISES

It is essential for older citizens who are controlling gout to participate in regular physical exercise. An individual's general well-being may be improved by performing straightforward exercises that are specifically designed to target particular areas of joint health, muscular strength, cardiovascular fitness, and flexibility. Throughout this chapter, we will investigate a wide selection of straightforward exercises for gout, which may be broken down into four distinct categories: range of motion activities, strengthening exercises, aerobic workouts, and flexibility exercises.

Range of Motion Exercises

For those who have gout, maintaining a complete range of motion in the joints is crucial since stiffness and decreased mobility are frequent symptoms both during and in between gout attacks. You may include a range of motion exercises into your regular regimen to assist develop joint flexibility.

- **Ankle Circles**

Ankle circles are easy exercises that help increase ankle flexibility.

1. With your feet flat on the floor, take a comfortable seat in a chair.

2. Raise one foot a little off the ground, then spend ten to fifteen seconds rotating your ankle clockwise.

3. Rotate your ankle in the other way for ten to fifteen seconds.

4. On the opposite ankle, repeat.

5. Several times a day, work on your ankle mobility with this drill.

- **Wrist Flexor and Extensor Stretch**

This exercise, which may be performed while seated, helps to maintain wrist flexibility.

1. Put your right arm out in front of you, palm down.

2. Apply a little pressure on your right hand's fingers with your left hand.

3. Hold for 15 to 30 seconds while noticing the forearm and wrist stretches.

4. Repeat with the other hand after switching.

5. Regularly perform this stretch to increase wrist range of motion.

- **Knee Flexion and Extension**

Exercises that involve knee flexion and extension help to increase knee joint flexibility.

- With your feet flat on the floor, take a seat on a chair's edge.

- Bring your right knee up to your chest as you slowly raise it off the ground.

- After a few seconds of holding still, straighten your leg.

- Proceed with the left leg.

- For each leg, do ten to fifteen repetitions, escalating the number as your comfort and strength permit.

- **Shoulder Circles**

Shoulder circles assist in preserving the shoulder joints' suppleness.

1. Put your arms down by your sides and take a comfortable stance or position.

2. Circularly, slowly raise your shoulders toward your ears.

3. After ten to fifteen seconds of continuous circular motion, reverse.

4. Regularly complete this exercise to release tension and improve shoulder range of motion.

Strengthening Exercises

Exercises that build muscle are essential for supporting gout-affected joints. Although it's important to use caution to prevent overdoing it, adding mild strengthening exercises to a regimen can improve joint health in general.

- **Leg Raises**

Leg raises may be modified to meet different fitness levels and help develop the thigh muscles.

1. With one leg bent and the other straight, lie on your back.

2. Maintaining the leg straight, raise it toward the ceiling.

3. Hold it for a little while before lowering it again so that it doesn't come into contact with the earth.

4. Perform ten to fifteen repetitions on each leg.

5. You may also perform this exercise while sitting on the edge of a chair if lying down is difficult.

- **Wall Push-Ups**

An easy method to build upper body strength is with wall push-ups.

1. With your hands at shoulder height and your palms against the wall, take a stance facing a wall.

2. Bend your elbows as you pull your chest closer to the wall while you lean towards it.

3. Return to the starting position by pushing.

4. Do ten to fifteen repetitions, escalating the number as your strength increases.

- **Seated Leg Press**

This sitting exercise can help build stronger muscles in your thighs.

1. With your feet flat on the floor and your back straight, take a seat on a firm chair.

2. Raise one leg straight out in front of you, keep it there for a little while, and then bring it back down.

3. Perform ten to fifteen repetitions on each leg.

4. Use resistance bands or ankle weights to enhance the resistance.

▪ **Bicep Curls with Light Weights**

You may utilize household objects or modest weights to strengthen your biceps.

1. Grab a little object with both hands (or use household items like water bottles).

2. Bend your elbows slightly to bring the weights closer to your shoulders while keeping your arms at your sides.

3. Return to the starting position with the weights lowered.

4. As your strength increases, progressively increase the number of repetitions to 10 to 15.

Cardiovascular Exercises

Exercises that involve the heart are vital for both general fitness and cardiac health. Low-impact activities are advised for elders with gout to reduce joint stress.

- **Brisk Walking**

A great low-impact cardiovascular workout is brisk walking.

1. Select a level, level area to walk on.

2. Warm up slowly at first, then progressively pick up the speed to a brisk walk.

3. Try to walk for at least 150 minutes a week at a moderate pace, or as your doctor may recommend.

4. If going outside is difficult for you, think about walking on a treadmill or through a mall.

- **Stationary Cycling**

The cardiovascular advantages of stationary cycling are achieved without compromising joint health.

1. For even more comfort, try riding a recumbent or stationary bike.
2. Warm up first, and then pedal at a comfortable speed.
3. Increase the resistance progressively for a harder exercise.
4. Each cycling session should last 30 minutes, with intensity adjustments as necessary.

- **Swimming or Water Aerobics**

Water aerobics and swimming are great options for cardiovascular workouts.

1. Swim comfortably, varying the effort according to your level of fitness.
2. Classes in water aerobics offer a regimented, joint-friendly exercise.
3. Water's buoyancy gives you a full-body workout while lessening the strain on your joints.

- **Dancing**

Getting your heart rate up may be enjoyable and beneficial when you dance.

1. Select dance forms like line dancing or ballroom dancing that have less impactful motions.

2. Learn dancing moves at home or enroll in a senior dance class.

3. Include dancing in your exercise regimen for a fun cardio workout.

Flexibility Exercises

For those with gout, maintaining flexibility is essential to preventing stiffness and improving joint health in general. Adding flexibility exercises to your program will help you move more freely.

▪ Yoga for Joint Flexibility

Yoga is a comprehensive, gentle exercise that improves joint flexibility.

1. Select yoga positions like Downward Dog, Child's Pose, and Cat-Cow that emphasize moderate stretches.

2. Regular yoga practice will increase flexibility and encourage calm.

3. Make adjustments to positions according to personal comfort by using supports like yoga blocks or straps.

- **Tai Chi for Balance and Flexibility**

Tai chi promotes flexibility and balance by combining slow, deliberate breathing with mild motions.

1. Follow senior-specific Tai Chi exercises that focus on slow, deliberate movements.

2. Take Tai Chi classes or utilize the internet tutorials.

3. Flexibility and joint health are often enhanced with tai chi.

- **Static Stretching for Muscle Flexibility**

Static stretching is a regular exercise that improves muscular flexibility.

1. Pay attention to your main muscle groups, such as your arms, legs, and back.
2. To improve relaxation, hold each stretch for 15 to 30 seconds while taking deep breaths.
3. Stretching with no movement should be done after warming up or as part of your cool-down.

- **Pilates for Core Strength and Flexibility**

Pilates uses exercises that improve flexibility and core strength.

1. Select Pilates poses that focus on deliberate stretches and motions.

2. Regular Pilates practice will enhance your general flexibility and stability of the core.

3. To add variation to your workouts, use Pilates props like stability balls or resistance bands.

CHAPTER FIVE: LIFESTYLE CHANGES

Reducing the symptoms of gout requires more than simply physical activity; it requires taking a comprehensive strategy that includes making adjustments to one's way of life. In this chapter, we will discuss some of the most important lifestyle adjustments that can have a favorable influence on the management of gout. The necessity of water in preventing gout episodes, the impact of sleep and stress management on general well-being, and dietary advice that is specifically customized for gout are some of the changes that are included in these modifications.

Dietary Tips for Gout Management

Diet is very important for controlling gout since some meals can aggravate the condition or make it go away. Elevated blood uric acid levels are linked to gout, which causes urate crystals to develop in the joints. Modifications in eating patterns can lower uric acid levels and lessen the frequency and intensity of gout episodes.

- **Limit Purine-Rich Foods**

Some meals include purines, which are substances that decompose into uric acid. Restricting the consumption of foods high in purines is necessary to manage gout by preventing the overproduction of uric acid. Purine-rich foods include:

- Organ meats: Meats from the liver, kidney, and other organs have a high purine content.

- Seafood: Fish that are high in purines include anchovies, mackerel, sardines, and shellfish.

- Red meat: Elevated uric acid levels have been linked to beef, lamb, and pig.

Moderation is crucial, even if certain items don't have to be completely avoided. A diet that prioritizes lean protein sources and allows for the occasional, rather than frequent, intake of foods high in purines, may be beneficial for seniors suffering from gout.

- **Increase Intake of Low-Fat Dairy**

Dairy products low in fat, such as yogurt and skim milk, have been linked to a decreased incidence of gout. Dairy products may aid in the body's uric acid excretion. Low-fat dairy products are recommended for seniors to eat to help control their gout. This can be as simple as having a serving of milk, yogurt, or another low-fat dairy product every day.

- **Choose Plant-Based Proteins**

Purines are often found in smaller amounts in plant-based proteins than in animal-based proteins. For elderly people with gout, increasing their intake of plant-based protein sources such as beans, tofu, and nuts may be helpful. Additional health advantages of plant-based proteins include fiber and a variety of vital minerals.

- **Stay Hydrated with Water**

Maintaining adequate hydration is crucial for managing gout. Drinking enough water lowers the body's high uric acid levels and lowers the chance of crystal development in the joints. Gouty seniors should try to consume 8 cups (64 ounces) of water a day, or as prescribed by their physician.

- **Limit Alcohol Intake, Especially Beer**

It is well known that alcohol, especially beer, raises uric acid levels and can aggravate gout episodes. Elderly people with gout are recommended to restrict their alcohol intake, with a focus on lowering their beer intake. For some people, moderate alcohol use may be okay, but for tailored advice, it's important to speak with a healthcare professional.

- **Maintain a Healthy Weight**

Since excess body weight is linked to increased uric acid production and decreased excretion, obesity is a major risk factor for gout. It is recommended that seniors maintain a healthy weight by combining regular physical exercise with a balanced diet. Not only may weight control help with gout treatment, but it also improves general health.

- **Consider Vitamin C Supplementation**

Less uric acid and a lower chance of gout episodes have been linked to vitamin C. Seniors who are high in vitamin C can think about including foods like bell peppers, citrus fruits, and strawberries in their diet. Healthcare professionals may occasionally advise vitamin C supplementation; however, this should only be carried out with expert advice.

Hydration and its Role in Gout Prevention

A key component of gout prevention is staying hydrated. A healthy diet and hydration routine support renal function at its peak, facilitating the body's effective excretion of uric acid. Conversely, dehydration raises the possibility of crystal formation in the joints by causing concentrated uric acid in the urine. In managing gout, keep in mind these crucial factors regarding hydration:

- **Drink Plenty of Water**

The greatest option for staying hydrated is water, particularly for gout sufferers. Elderly people should try to consume 8 cups (64 ounces) of water or more each day, spaced out throughout the day. Drinking water regularly promotes the body's natural process of removing uric acid through the urine and helps one stay hydrated.

- **Limit Sugary and Caffeinated Beverages**

Sugar-filled drinks, such as sodas and some fruit juices, may exacerbate the symptoms of gout. Dehydration is another side effect of high coffee use. Gout-affected seniors should limit their intake of sugar-filled and caffeinated drinks and, if at all feasible, stick to water as their main hydration option.

- **Include Hydrating Foods**

A few meals can help you stay hydrated overall because of their high water content. Fruits and vegetables high in water, such as oranges, cucumbers, and watermelon, can make tasty additions to the diet. Consuming these hydrated meals enhances the advantages of drinking water.

- **Monitor Urine Color**

Urine color monitoring can reveal information about hydration levels. While dark yellow or amber-colored urine may suggest dehydration, clear or light yellow pee usually indicates adequate hydration. It is advised for seniors to monitor the color of their urine and modify their fluid intake as necessary.

▪ **Be Mindful of Alcohol's Dehydrating Effects**

Drinking alcohol might make you more dehydrated, which can make your gout symptoms worse. Elderly people with gout should exercise caution when it comes to drinking alcohol and make sure they are getting enough water, especially if they do.

Sleep and Stress Management

In addition to being essential to general wellbeing, getting enough sleep and managing stress are also key to managing gout. Chronic stress and inadequate sleep have both been related to elevated inflammatory levels and may be initiators of gout episodes. Here are some things to think about to maximize sleep and reduce stress:

- **Prioritize Quality Sleep**

Good sleep has a favorable effect on managing gout and is crucial for general health. It is advised for seniors to develop sound sleeping practices, such as:

- Maintain a Regular Sleep Schedule: The body's internal clock is regulated when bedtime and wake-up times are the same each day.

- Comfy Sleep Environment: Having a cozy and accommodating sleeping space, complete with cushions and a comfortable mattress, helps promote sound sleep.

- Reducing Stimulants: You can improve the quality of your sleep by avoiding electronics and coffee just before bed.

- **Incorporate Relaxation Techniques**

Gout symptoms may be exacerbated by ongoing stress. To properly manage stress, seniors are recommended to include relaxation practices in their daily routine. Stress can be decreased and a sense of calm can be fostered by practices including progressive muscle relaxation, deep breathing, and meditation.

- **Stay Active for Stress Relief**

Beyond its benefits for managing gout, regular physical exercise also helps lower stress levels. Walking, yoga, and tai chi are examples of exercises that can improve one's physical and mental health. It is recommended that seniors engage in enjoyable and soothing activities.

- **Seek Social Support**

Keeping up social ties and asking friends and relatives for help might help give emotional support when things get tough. The promotion of healthy social relationships, discussing worries, and exchanging personal experiences all enhance general well-being.

▪ Consider Professional Support

Seniors who experience extreme stress may want to think about getting help from a specialist. Psychologists and counselors who specialize in mental health issues can offer coping mechanisms for handling stress and emotional difficulties. Personalized advice can also result from open conversations about stresses with healthcare practitioners.

CHAPTER SIX: REAL-LIFE SUCCESS STORIES

In this chapter, we look into the motivational real-life success tales of older citizens who have successfully managed their gout via the use of exercise, their ability to overcome obstacles and the celebration of their accomplishments. These stories shed light on the transformational effect of taking a comprehensive approach to the management of gout, which includes engaging in regular physical activity that is adapted to the specific requirements and capabilities of each individual being treated.

Inspiring Accounts of Seniors Managing Gout Through Exercise

A multimodal approach is typically used to treat gout, and exercise is essential for promoting joint health, lowering inflammation, and boosting general wellbeing. The following true success stories show how seniors have overcome gout-related obstacles by making exercise a regular part of their lives.

Sarah's Journey to Joint Health:

The 68-year-old Sarah was given a gout diagnosis a few years ago. Having to deal with joint discomfort and restricted movement, she decided to exercise to manage her health. Sarah began with low-impact exercises like regular walks and light stretching. She eventually began utilizing resistance bands for resistance training under the supervision of her physical therapist to strengthen the muscles that supported her joints.

Sarah's experience is unique because of her dedication to consistency. She began with brief workouts and progressively increased the length and intensity of her regimen. By enrolling in a neighborhood senior exercise class, Sarah was able to connect with others her age and gain support from others going through similar struggles.

In addition to successfully managing her gout today, Sarah reports increases in her general level of energy and fitness. She is proof of the life-changing potential of individualized fitness regimens catered to each person's capabilities and medical background.

John's Rediscovery of Mobility:

John was seventy-two years old and had both arthritis and gout, which limited his movement. John was determined to restore his freedom, so he started an aquatic workout regimen to find mobility. John found that swimming and water aerobics were low-impact, efficient ways to increase muscular strength and joint flexibility without overstressing his joints.

John's secret to success is that he discovered an exercise regimen that satisfied him emotionally as well as his bodily needs. His motions were aided by the buoyancy of the water, which made the exercises easier to do and more fun. Regular swimming lessons under the guidance of an experienced teacher were a vital component of John's gout treatment plan.

John's quality of life improved gradually as he had more joint mobility, less discomfort, and overall improvement. His experience serves as a reminder of the value of experimenting with different forms of exercise to determine which suits personal tastes and medical needs the best.

Mary's Journey from Sedentary to Active:

When Mary, 75, was diagnosed with gout, she had been living a largely sedentary lifestyle. When Mary realized she needed to make adjustments to her lifestyle, she went into the process with a realistic and methodical attitude. She began by taking modest strolls in her neighborhood, and as her endurance increased, she progressively went farther.

Mary's tale is noteworthy because of her dedication to moving a part of her everyday life. Mary came up with inventive methods to be active rather than thinking of exercise as a distinct pastime. She joined a gardening club in her community so that she could take care of her garden and do some light exercise. Mary also learned the advantages of chair exercises, which helped her strengthen her joints and muscles while seated.

Mary developed a fresh passion for an active lifestyle in addition to efficiently managing her gout via persistent effort and a willingness to adapt. Seniors who are considering making the switch from a sedentary to an active lifestyle might find encouragement in her narrative.

These true success stories demonstrate the variety of approaches people may take when using exercise to manage gout. Personalized ways that matched their talents, interests, and health problems were discovered by these elders, whether it was by walking, chair exercises, or water aerobics. Their experiences highlight how crucial customized exercise regimens, perseverance, and an optimistic outlook are to successful gout management.

Overcoming Challenges and Celebrating Achievements

Exercise-based gout management is not without its difficulties, even if the path is frequently filled with success. Gout-affected seniors may face challenges that call for tenacity, flexibility, and a strong support system. The experiences that follow demonstrate the tenacity of people who overcome obstacles and achieve noteworthy accomplishments on their road toward managing gout.

Tom's Resilience in the Face of Flare-Ups:

Gout flare-ups became a problem for 70-year-old Tom, who loved hiking and found it difficult to continue his active lifestyle. Tom worked hard with his healthcare team to establish tactics for controlling flare-ups while continuing his busy lifestyle, refusing to give in to frustration.

Tom modified his workout regimen to include calming activities like swimming or stationary cycling during episodes of severe gout symptoms since they reduced the strain on his afflicted joints. He also developed an awareness of his body's cues, which enabled him to adjust his exercise regimen in response to the intensity of his symptoms.

Tom overcame obstacles without compromising his dedication to an athletic lifestyle because of his tenacity and flexibility. Through collaboration with his medical professionals and deliberate modifications, Tom maintained his enjoyment of his favorite physical pursuits.

Grace's Support System and Accountability:

The 73-year-old grandma Grace was having trouble maintaining her workout schedule. Grace found it difficult to keep going because of the responsibilities of everyday life and her sporadic painful episodes. Seeing that she needed assistance, she called on her relatives.

Grace's grandkids took an interest in exercise and began going on walks with her and doing modest exercises at home. In addition to making the events more fun, having a support structure in place also gave people a sense of responsibility. Grace discovered that her dedication to maintaining an active lifestyle turned into a family project.

Grace acknowledged and appreciated both her accomplishments and the beneficial effects of her trip on her family's health despite the ups and downs. Her experience highlights the need to have a strong social network to help one overcome obstacles and develop a feeling of responsibility when trying to treat gout with exercise.

Robert's Gradual Progress and Patience:

When Robert, 68, started using exercise as a way to control his gout, he had to deal with impatience. He first pushed himself too hard since he was eager to see results quickly, which compounded his agony and dissatisfaction. Robert changed his strategy to be more patient and progressive after realizing the value of pacing oneself.

Robert carefully collaborated with his physical therapist to create a personalized training regimen that put joint health and steady advancement first. He recognized that sustained growth frequently requires patience and appreciated modest victories, such as improved flexibility and decreased discomfort during exercise.

The lesson from Robert's tale is that managing gout with exercise is a marathon, not a sprint. People can surmount obstacles and attain long-lasting enhancements in their joint health by adopting a patient and cautious approach.

CHAPTER SEVEN: FREQUENTLY ASKED QUESTIONS

When it comes to gout management via exercise, older citizens frequently discover that they have several questions. The purpose of this chapter is to address frequent concerns regarding exercise and gout and to provide answers and guidance from experts in order to empower individuals on their road toward joint health.

Common Concerns About Exercise and Gout

• *Can Exercise Trigger Gout Attacks?*

This is a typical worry for gout sufferers, since they may refrain from exercising out of fear of inciting excruciating bouts. Nonetheless, it's generally accepted that frequent, moderate exercise helps treat gout. While high-impact and high-intensity workouts may be dangerous during acute flare-ups, customized exercise regimens, and low-impact pursuits can improve joint health without aggravating symptoms.

It's critical to collaborate closely with medical providers and tailor workout regimens to the severity of gout symptoms as well as individual demands. A gradual increase in intensity, suitable warm-ups, and adjustments made during flare-ups might reduce the likelihood of gout episodes brought on by activity.

- ***What Kinds of Exercise Are Good for Gouty Seniors?***

Gouty seniors are advised to take part in a range of activities that support joint health without putting undue strain on their afflicted joints. Walking, swimming, stationary cycling, and light stretching are examples of low-impact exercises that are frequently advantageous and well-tolerated. These exercises improve general wellbeing, strengthen supporting muscles, and increase flexibility.

Exercise regimens must be customized to each person's talents, interests, and current medical issues. Creating individualized exercise programs that meet the unique requirements of geriatric gout patients can be made easier by collaborating with healthcare professionals like physical therapists or fitness specialists.

- **How Can Gout Flare-Ups Affect Seniors' Ability to Stay Active?**

While flare-ups might be difficult, an active lifestyle shouldn't be entirely derailed by them. Exercise regimens should be adjusted to suit the afflicted joints during acute bouts. During flare-ups, low-impact exercises like stationary cycling, water aerobics, and mild stretching are frequently well tolerated.

It's critical to pay attention to your body's cues and modify the type and intensity of exercise as necessary. Even when gout symptoms are worse, seniors can stay active by consulting with healthcare specialists about appropriate adjustments and adding joint-friendly activities.

- ***Are Seniors with Gout Safe to Perform Strength Training?***

For elders with gout, strength exercises can be safe and helpful when done properly and under supervision. Increasing muscular strength can help to maintain joint stability and promote better joint health in general. Strength training must be done carefully, though, particularly in the event of severe flare-ups.

Creating a personalized strength training program with the assistance of a physical therapist or fitness specialist is advised. Seniors can safely increase strength by beginning with low-resistance activities and then increasing the intensity. Safe strength training also involves correct warm-ups and cool-downs, as well as making sure that there is enough recovery in between sessions.

- ***Can Physical Activity Help Lower Gout Medication Dependency?***

Exercise is essential for managing gout, but it cannot take the place of medical care. Prescription drugs from medical professionals are crucial for lowering inflammation, managing uric acid levels, and averting gout outbreaks. Exercise enhances general well-being, improves flexibility, and supports joint health in addition to medicine.

Seniors shouldn't try to rely only on exercise to substitute prescription drugs. Rather, they have to collaborate with their medical team to create a thorough treatment plan that incorporates the right kind of activity as well as medicine.

Expert Answers and Advice

- ***What Function Does a Physical Therapist Serve in the Treatment of Gout?***

Physical therapists offer individualized exercise regimens and advice, which is a big part of their involvement in managing gout. They evaluate how well joints function, treat muscle imbalances, and create training plans that maximize strength and mobility while reducing strain on injured joints. Seniors can learn from physical therapists about assistive technology, good body mechanics, and movement-based gout treatment techniques.

Working together with a physical therapist guarantees that workout regimens are safe, efficient, and tailored to each person's requirements. Maintaining regular contact with the medical staff enables modifications to the workout regimen based on the patient's development and any changes in their health.

- ***How Can Fitness Professionals Assist Gouty Seniors?***

Professionals with certification in fitness, such as senior fitness specialists in personal training, can be of great assistance in managing gout. Exercise regimens created by fitness professionals take into account each person's talents, interests, and medical circumstances.

They provide changes, assess progress, and mentor elders in executing exercises with appropriate techniques.

Working with fitness professionals adds diversity to workout regimens, which keeps older adults interested and involved. Fitness instructors may also improve the general health of elders by encouraging a happy and encouraging environment during exercise.

- ***Do Seniors with Gout Get Special Treatment in Group Exercise Classes?***

Group fitness sessions can be beneficial for seniors suffering from gout, as long as certain precautions are taken. Instructors must be cognizant of each participant's unique requirements and any accommodations needed to manage gout. Group exercises that emphasize low-impact activities, such as water aerobics or senior aerobics, are typically a good fit for those with gout.

Seniors should discuss their condition and any necessary special accommodations with their teachers. Selecting programs taught by teachers knowledgeable in senior exercise is advised. If at all feasible, let the instructors know about any current flare-ups or symptoms of gout.

- ***What Role Does a Rheumatologist Play in the Management of Gout?***

Specialist physicians in the field of rheumatology, known as rheumatologists, are essential in the care of gout. They identify gout, evaluate how severe it is, and recommend drugs to lower uric acid levels and treat symptoms. To create all-encompassing treatment programs, rheumatologists collaborate with physical therapists and fitness specialists in addition to other medical professionals.

Consulting a rheumatologist regularly makes it possible to continuously assess gout treatment plans. They could change prescriptions, offer advice on changing one's lifestyle, and deal with any new gout-related issues.

• *Can Gout Be Managed by Dietary Adjustments Alone Without Exercise?*

Although dietary modifications are a crucial part of managing gout, they work best when paired with consistent exercise and medicinal intervention. Controlling uric acid levels requires a balanced diet that includes water, moderates purine-rich foods, and promotes general health.

Exercise prevents stiffness, supports weight control, and improves joint health in addition to dietary modifications. A balanced diet, consistent exercise, and prescription drugs work together to give a holistic strategy for controlling gout and lowering the frequency and intensity of gout episodes.

CONCLUSION

As we get to the end of this extensive guide on "Simple Gout Exercises for Seniors," it is crucial to reflect on the most important lessons and urge elderly citizens to adopt a lifestyle that is more active and healthier. In the chapters that came before this one, we discussed the complexities of gout, including the significance of workouts, the alterations that should be made to one's lifestyle, success stories, and the opinions of specialists. It is the purpose of this final chapter to summarize the most important lessons learned and to encourage elderly citizens to make well-informed decisions that will improve their overall health.

Recap of Key Takeaways

Comprehending Senior Gout.

One of the main symptoms of gout, an inflammatory arthritis that affects the joints, is abrupt, intense flare-ups of pain, swelling, and redness. Gout is more common among seniors because of age, gender, heredity, and lifestyle choices. Comprehending the fundamental reasons and indications of gout is essential for efficient handling.

Exercise is Crucial for Gout Management.

An essential component of geriatric gout therapy is exercise. Frequent exercise has several advantages, such as better joint health, more flexibility, stronger muscles, and general well-being. Exercises with low impact that are customized for each person are essential for lowering the frequency and intensity of gout attacks.

Fundamentals of Gout.

Understanding the disease, its origins, risk factors, symptoms, and the diagnostic procedure are all important components of learning the fundamentals of gout. Seniors may collaborate with healthcare experts to create efficient plans for symptom management and prevention by learning more about the causes of gout.

Gout and exercise.

Examining the connection between exercise and gout, we looked at the advantages of physical activity for elderly people with gout. Exercise provides a comprehensive approach to managing gout by improving joint flexibility and cardiovascular health. The necessity of regular physical activity, types of exercises, and things to think about before beginning an exercise plan were all covered.

Customizing Senior Exercise Programs.

Senior exercise routines should be tailored to their specific needs by working with healthcare providers, knowing the difference between high- and low-impact activities, and meeting their needs. The need for customized exercise regimens to optimize benefits and reduce the chance of aggravating gout symptoms was highlighted in this chapter.

Simple Gout Exercises.

We divided the exercises into four categories: range of motion, strengthening, cardiovascular, and flexibility in our investigation of basic gout exercises. Seniors have a wide variety of activities to select from, including walking, yoga, bicep curls, and ankle circles, enabling them to create pleasurable and customized regimens.

Adjusting Your Lifestyle to Manage Your Gout.

A holistic approach to managing gout requires a lifestyle change, which includes nutrition advice, staying hydrated, getting enough sleep, and managing stress. An overall plan for managing gout symptoms includes balancing purine-rich meals with low-fat dairy, drinking enough water, getting enough sleep, and using stress-reduction tactics.

Success Stories from Real Life.

Moving stories of elderly people effectively controlling their gout with exercise demonstrated the transformational potential of taking a comprehensive approach. These tales showed the resiliency, flexibility, and persistence of people in conquering obstacles, from regaining mobility through water aerobics to progressively increasing strength training.

Encouragement for a Healthier, Active Lifestyle

- **Embracing Personalized Wellness**

As elders begin their road to gout control with exercise, it is critical to acknowledge the individuality of each person's situation. Personalized health is understanding one's own body, recognizing personal limits, and adjusting lifestyle choices to meet individual needs.

Working collaboratively with healthcare specialists such as rheumatologists, physical therapists, and fitness experts ensures that gout management tactics are precise. Regular communication and feedback allow for modifications, which improve the efficacy of fitness programs and lifestyle improvements.

- ***Exercise's Overall Benefits.***

Exercise is more than just a duty to do; it is a dynamic and transformational journey that promotes physical, mental, and emotional health. Seniors are taught to see exercise as a comprehensive discipline that goes beyond the physical rewards. Engaging in enjoyable activities, such as a nature walk, a dancing class, or a mild yoga practice, helps to maintain a good mentality and emotional resilience.

Exercise has a positive overall benefit, including better sleep, lower stress levels, greater mood, and a sense of accomplishment. Seniors may establish a long-term and joyful connection with physical activity by recognizing and enjoying its many advantages.

- ***Celebrating both big and little achievements.***

Celebrating achievement is essential while striving for a better, more active lifestyle. Every stride taken, stretch finished, and milestone accomplished is a reason to celebrate. Seniors are encouraged to recognize and appreciate both major and small accomplishments during their journey.

The road to gout control may be difficult, and progress may take time. Seniors may create a happy and resilient attitude by adopting a mentality that appreciates both the trip and the outcome. Celebrating progress boosts motivation and supports the desire for long-term well-being.

- ***Building a supportive community.***

The value of a supporting community cannot be understated. Fostering a supportive community, whether via group exercise classes, family activities, or interacting with people experiencing similar issues, promotes a sense of belonging and drive.

Sharing one's experiences, struggles, and accomplishments with others helps to build an encouraging network. Seniors are urged to seek out local and online communities that share their interests and ambitions. The combined support of a community improves the entire path to gout control through exercise.

- ***Embracing lifelong learning.***

Pursuing a healthier, more active lifestyle is an ongoing learning experience. Seniors are urged to embrace their curiosity, try new activities, and remain up to date on developments in gout management and senior fitness. Learning about the most recent research, exercise routines, and wellness practices enables people to make educated decisions that meet their changing requirements.

Lifelong learning promotes a sense of empowerment. Seniors may actively shape their well-being by remaining inquiring, seeking information, and being open to new ideas in the realms of gout treatment and exercise.

Closing Thoughts

In summary, treating gout in seniors with easy workouts is a comprehensive approach to enjoying life to the fullest, not simply a health tactic. Seniors may go beyond symptom treatment by learning about the nuances of gout, adopting individualized fitness regimens, changing their lifestyles, and finding motivation from real-life success stories.

Every page that seniors turn in their lives is a chance to celebrate the freedom of movement, the body's tenacity, and the possibility of further development and well-being. Seniors may control their gout via exercise dynamically and powerfully, one step at a time, and closer

to a joyful, active, and healthier living.

APPENDIX

Providing sample workout regimens that are specifically designed for older citizens who are managing gout and offering extra resources to help their path toward optimal joint health are both included in the appendix, which acts as a great resource section.

Sample Exercise Plans

1 Week 1-4: Gentle Movement and Flexibility

Day 1-3: Walking Routine

- Warm-up (5 minutes): Do some light wrist stretches and ankle circles.

- The main activity for fifteen minutes is brisk walking in a level, safe location or around the neighborhood.

- Stretching lightly for the thighs, wrists, and calves is the cool-down (5 minutes).

Day 4: Rest or Gentle Yoga

- Five minutes of deep breathing exercises to warm up.

- Main Activity (20 minutes): Mild yoga postures with an emphasis on joint mobility and flexibility.

- 5 minutes of guided relaxation and light stretching to wind down.

Day 5-7: Low-Impact Aerobics

- Warm-up: Do a quick aerobic warm-up, such as marching in place, for five minutes.

- Main Activity (20 minutes): Arm motions, knee lifts, and side steps as part of a low-impact aerobics program.

- Five minutes of slow motion and stretching to cool down.

Week 5-8: Strength Building and Cardiovascular Health

Day 1-3: Strength Training.

- Warm-up: Light aerobic warm-up, such as brisk cycling or marching, for five minutes.

- Strength exercise with resistance bands or small weights is the main activity (20 minutes). Pay attention to your main muscle groups, such as your arms, legs, and core.

- After five minutes of cooling down, gently stretch the affected muscles.

Day 4: Rest or Water Aerobics

- Warm-up (5 minutes): Light water motions or strolling in the water.

- The main activity lasts for twenty minutes and consists of a water aerobics program with arm and leg motions.

- Cool Down (5 minutes): Take a relaxing dip in the water or practice floating.

Day 5-7: Cardiovascular Exercise

- 5 minutes of vigorous walking or cycling for a warm-up.

- Main Activity (20 minutes): Cardiovascular activity at a moderate level, including riding an elliptical machine, swimming, or cycling.

- Cool Down (5 minutes): Light stretching and strolling at a leisurely pace.

Week 9-12: Flexibility and Endurance

Day 1-3: Flexibility Focus

- Five minutes of warm-up: joint mobility movements, such as light wrist, ankle, and shoulder circles.

- Main Exercise (20 minutes): Balance and flexibility are the focus of a yoga or pilates class.

- 5 minutes of guided relaxation and exercises to cool down.

Day 4: Rest or Gentle Cardio

- Warm-up: Light aerobic exercises, such as stationary cycling or marching in place, should take five minutes.

- Main Activity: Low-impact cardiovascular exercise with an emphasis on steady-state movement (20 minutes).

- Five minutes of slow motion and stretching to cool down.

Day 5-7: Endurance Building

- Warm-up (5 minutes): Light exercise or brisk walking.

- Main Activity (25 minutes): Vigor-focused activity, such as slow-paced cycling or longer walks.

- Cool down (5 minutes): Light stretching and strolling at a leisurely pace.

These exemplary fitness regimens are made to be flexible enough to accommodate personal preferences and needs. It is essential to confer with medical professionals, like physical therapists or fitness specialists, to tailor these regimens according to individual medical conditions and gout control objectives.